"Alzheimer's: So That's What It's Going to Be"

Jim Bergstrom

By

Catherine Bergstrom

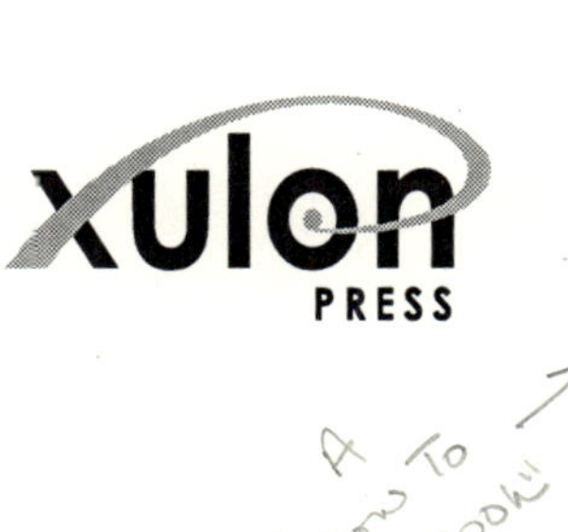

"Alzheimer's: So That's What It's Going to Be"
Jim Bergstrom
by Catherine Bergstrom

Printed in the United States of America

ISBN 9781626972575

www.xulonpress.com

Contents

Preface

More than once, while Jim could still express himself, he told his doctors and nurses, "I've had a wonderful life."

This story reflects but a small fraction of that life—after he was diagnosed with Alzheimer's. What I hope his story does reflect, especially for those who knew and loved him, is his character, in spite of the disease. He was not shy about his diagnosis and he approached it in a practical way while he still could.

I think if I could tell him that I was writing about his life with Alzheimer's he would say, "Go for it."

Dedication Page

This book is dedicated to all caregivers and to all the caregivers of caregivers who carry us throughout the difficult years of Alzheimer's.

PART I

Diagnosis Alzheimer's April 2006

An estimated 5.4 million Americans are
living with Alzheimer's disease.

Alzheimer's Association

Jim and I had errands to run that April morning in 2006, so we left the house separately, agreeing to meet at the doctor's office. The doctor was a neurologist and this was the last appointment after a series of tests that had been ordered: cognitive reasoning, brain scan, and blood work among others. Jim had made a decision to see a doctor some weeks before as he said he didn't seem able to do the things he wanted to, primarily giving tours at the National Air and Space Museum's Steven F. Udvar-Hazy Center where he had been a docent (tour guide) for 15 years.

The doctor was brief. He noted a deficit in Jim's cognitive reasoning, told us his diagnosis was early onset Alzheimer's, gave us prescriptions for some pills, did not elaborate about what to expect, mentioned something about two - four years, and told us to come back in a few months.

We didn't ask what two - four years meant. We just left and as we stood outside in front of the medical building, Jim said, "Alzheimer's. So that's what it's going to be," and he left to go out to the museum, his home away from home.

And that is the abruptness with which this fearful disease entered our lives, and I say "our lives" because for every Alzheimer's patient there is a caregiver. Alzheimer's: it wasn't a brain tumor, or a hearing problem, or some other disease for which there might be a cure. We had been married for 45 years, a positive shared time. I, too, had known something was wrong and close friends had been suggesting that Jim needed to see a doctor, but I had been reluctant to bring up the subject with Jim.

There were two instances in particular that rang alarm bells about Jim's thinking. The year before his diagnosis, we were invited to the wedding of a friend's son. The wedding was some distance from our familiar area, but we had a detailed map and instructions to follow. By this time I was doing most of the driving when we were together, and in daylight had followed the map easily. But the trip home was another matter. It was dark and Jim couldn't follow the map or directions in reverse. He just couldn't do it and finally I stopped and studied the map. I say it was shocking to me as Jim had flown Navy aircraft in numerous places around the world, over vast oceans, and always managed to find the carrier or an airfield to land. It was also shocking as he wasn't frustrated by his present inability to find his way. He was like a child just expecting me to know.

The other incident that should have been an eye opener for me happened on a visit with my family in Colorado. We were all enjoying a dominos game and asked Jim to join us, but he wasn't able to follow the rules or even distinguish the different tiles. This, from a man who was a very good card player and had enjoyed other more complicated games as well. Though all of us who were playing dominos were suddenly aware of his "loss', he didn't seem to notice.

Even five years before his diagnosis, I had made the comment to my sons-in-law that if anything happened to me, Jim shouldn't stay in the house alone. He was extremely focused on the projects he was working on at the museum, but didn't bother about much else; I used the expression "slip-sliding" away" to describe his behavior.

So the diagnosis of Alzheimer's based on lack of cognitive reasoning skill was not a surprise. Jim seemed to accept it with equanimity and he didn't try to keep it a secret. He just went about doing what he loved, no longer giving tours, but focusing on putting a library together for the new museum. The library would be a reference room for the docents to use—information about all the aircraft.

Looking back on that day of the diagnosis, it surprised me how calmly we both took the news, but Jim and I had already experienced the greatest loss and trauma imaginable to us: the loss of our son. David, a naval aviator, was killed when his Navy jet crashed at an air show in June, 2000. The pain and grief were devastating, but the experience of God's healing grace was transforming, and so whatever else happened in our lives, we knew trust in God's presence was essential.

Not long after Jim's diagnosis, my daughter, Karen, and I went to a book signing and talk about Alzheimer's at the Vienna Public Library. The author giving the talk, Frank Fuerst, had cared for his wife, who had Alzheimer's, for seventeen years. His book, *Alzheimer's—Care with Dignity*, was reviewed in the *Washington Post* and highly recommended.

I bought the book and that evening started reading it, but it was overwhelming reading for me, a beginner on this journey of dementia. I read halfway through the very detailed book before I put it aside and decided I would use it as a resource when needed. The book is excellent and if one has a question about almost anything related to the care of a loved one with Alzheimer's, it is answered there. Very practical.

His book, though, started me thinking. I like books and there are probably many caregivers (or potential caregivers) out there who would like another story, one with a different slant—not a "how to" book, but a story about an ordinary family and how they coped. Our experience is not everyone else's, and, as Maria Shriver commented in a TV special about

Alzheimer's, "Once you've seen one case of Alzheimer's, you've seen *one* case." Her father had Alzheimer's and while this disease has many stages, it is as different as people are different.

Unfortunately the commonality of the disease is that it is relentless in its downward spiral and eventually robs its victims of their lives.

Almost without fail, all of our acquaintances, when they learned Jim had Alzheimer's, wanted to know how it started… What were the signs? One could sense their worry—maybe their memory wasn't as good as it used to be. I would tell them that it wasn't losing or misplacing the car keys or glasses or whatever the item that mattered; it was not knowing what they were used for when you found them. My daughter, Patty, tells me the new buzz word is "partial-heimers."

But the larger worry is this tsunami that is about to overtake our society. In a strange way, though, this worry generates hope because the pressure is increasing to find the cause (and eventually prevention or cure). Numbers generate monies and research…I've already seen what the growing awareness has accomplished.

So I write this story, Jim's and mine, about the disease, caregivers, support groups, new facilities (day care, assisted living), human angels, and even our dog, Daisy, who is quite a companion. Even the daily emails I was sending to my family would become part of this story. I include clips of the emails sent to family during the last two years of "our life with Alzheimer's" in order to give depth and insight in various places throughout the book.

Public Awareness

My assumption is that the story of any one of us is in some measure the story of us all.

Frederick Buechner

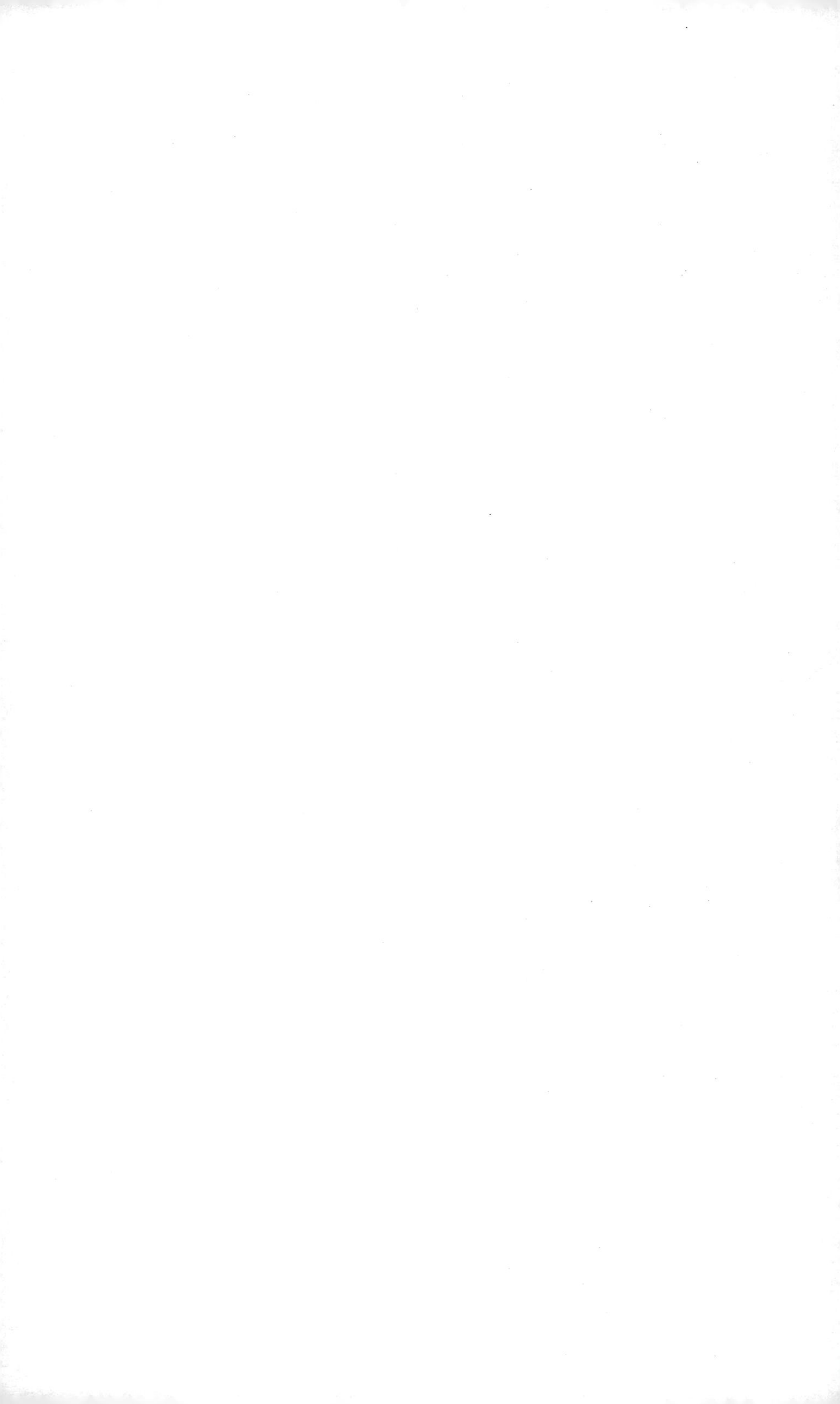

To my mind, public awareness and recognition of Alzheimer's really began when former President Reagan wrote a letter to the American people in 1994 revealing that he was suffering from Alzheimer's disease. Sandra Day O'Connor, the first female Supreme Court Justice, retired in 2006 citing the needs of her husband who had Alzheimer's disease. Both former President Reagan and Justice O'Connor deserve credit for their honesty about the disease. It opened the door and brought out for public discussion and action what so many had quietly struggled with for so long…as I had when I cared for Jim's mother, Hildur.

Hildur had come to live with us in the mid 1980's. She was recovering from a fall, had memory loss, and as I soon discovered, needed help with bathing, dressing, eating and couldn't be left alone. When she first moved from Arizona to live with us, I took her to our family doctor to establish her medical care; she had only a standard physical. Months later I made an appointment for her again as I hoped to get some assistance/direction/medication…I didn't know what! I was isolated. So was she with her failing abilities, and I wrote a letter for the doctor detailing all those. I wrote the letter as I didn't want to talk about her (and her loss) in front of her. I hoped the doctor would grasp the situation. Maybe there was a medication she could take.

But the doctor ignored my written comments, and asked her who was president of the United States. Well…she loved President Reagan so she gave the right answer, and I felt like the evil daughter-in-law trying to institutionalize a lovely old person when in reality I just wanted support. She was lovely and we had always been very close to one another. So we continued in our splendid isolation. The doctor was as ignorant as I was.

Even when Hildur lost consciousness one day and fell to the floor and I called 911 and had her taken to the Emergency Room…even then, the young doctor said she had a temporary passing light stroke and those were not uncommon in the elderly. Not to worry! In other words, don't call 911 should this happen again.

Once I hired a neighbor girl, a high school senior whom Hildur knew, to come stay with her while I ran errands. But Hildur became so angry and uncooperative that I didn't try that again.

Finally, Jim realized that I couldn't provide 24/7 care for his mom (I say finally as I've often observed denial on the part of family members who are not the full time caregivers… this can be adult children, spouses, and other extended family members.). Jim began looking at what was available for care for Hildur, which at the time were nursing homes. He chose the best one in our area, thinking his mom could live on the floor for "independent" residents, but it only took the staff about an hour to recognize she wasn't and couldn't be independent.

The nursing home administrator acknowledged the floor for "dementia" patients was not satisfactory. They had just put a kind of fence and gate across the end of one floor; no outside access, small double rooms, a noisy, institutional dining area, very limited activity—-mostly residents just sat in wheelchairs in front of the one large TV. It all just made me sad.

We visited Hildur often, and they did have a lovely large room on another floor where we could talk and enjoy pleasant surroundings. There was also a small but attractive garden seating area for visitors to use in good weather. The staff was caring and we often brought Hildur "home" to have dinner with us.

She never complained. But I see now that she would have thrived in a day care program or even as she needed more assistance, in an assisted living facility. Her long eight years in that nursing home still touches me with sadness.

Angels in Our Midst

Do not neglect to show hospitality to strangers,
For by this some have entertained angels
without knowing it.

Hebrews 13:2

Alzheimer's has become so prevalent that almost everyone we knew or met would say, "I have an aunt or uncle, a grandparent or parent or a neighbor who has Alzheimer's." So, they knew without asking when help was needed. They became the angels in our midst.

One summer day I happened to glance out the window just as a white SUV pulled into our driveway. In a few minutes, Jim came in the back door and told me that he had had a flat tire. I asked where the car was and he pulled a slip of paper from his pocket with the location of the car written on it. I was about to call AAA when the phone rang and the person who had driven Jim home was on the other end. She said she was driving on her street and saw an older man standing by his car… a flat tire. He looked confused and she noticed the military sticker on the windshield. The man reminded her of her dad so she stopped and offered to help by taking him home. I thanked her—-she never said her name and I wonder to this day how she knew exactly what needed to be done… writing down the location of the car…finding out where Jim lived and his phone number and calling me. How did she know Jim wouldn't remember where the car was, that she should write it down. Maybe she was remembering her dad.

Another day, Jim was out walking, which he enjoyed doing, and after a while the door bell rang. It was Jim with a neighbor from a few blocks over. Apparently this neighbor, who knew Jim from their work together on the neighborhood parks committee years before, saw Jim walking almost in circles and realized something was wrong. Jim was confused and so the neighbor walked home with him. I thanked him and was holding the door open for Jim to come inside. But Jim turned and started to walk away. I asked where he was going. "Home," he said and wouldn't accept that he was home. So I said, "Okay, but first come in and have lunch." He accepted that. So much for going for walks alone, and I began to understand that "home" had taken on a new meaning for Jim. I also recognized that not arguing, but just changing the subject was the easiest way to cope.

Once, on an errand to Target with Jim, he disappeared after saying he was going to look for gloves. I started looking up and down the aisle for him when a young clerk said, "He's in the aisle with tools." I thanked her and thought how observant she'd been to know who the object of my search was… or even that I was searching!

The most professional angel in our midst was Michelle, a nurse practitioner in the neurologist's office who was very kind, caring and knowledgeable, and she always spoke directly to Jim, taking as much time as needed. It was obvious that Jim trusted her and respected her comments. We saw her every three months, or more frequently as needed, until Jim moved into assisted living in June 2010.

But a driving excursion Jim had in February 2009 pushed me to realize we were over-taxing the angels.

One morning, Jim told me that one of his teeth had broken and it had, but our regular dentist was out of town so an appointment was made with his "stand-by," a dentist in a different location. Jim was still driving at this point and always left home a least an hour earlier—-he wanted to be on time he said. (Actually, as I discovered later, he often got lost and took extra time.) On this particular day, he left early and about two hours later, the phone rang. It was the secretary at the new dentist's office saying Jim hadn't arrived. She was so concerned when I told her he was headed there hours ago that she made me promise I'd call her when he got home. Another couple of hours passed and finally Jim pulled into the garage. He didn't know where he had been, but had numerous slips of paper in his pocket giving directions. I figured out from those slips of papers that he had been in the Baltimore area—a long way from our neighborhood in Northern Virginia! Obviously many people had tried to help him.

I called the dentist's office to say he was home. At this point, you, the reader, may wonder why Jim was driving at all, and writing this story, I ask myself the same question.

But Jim was always a very independent person, and we were at that stage in his disease where we still felt he could drive. It was one thing he held on to, and I was holding on to that also. I think everyone watching us—family and neighbors—were holding their collective breaths.

Eventually driving was no longer an option for Jim. One day he came home and told me that a policeman got angry with him. Naturally I asked what had happened. Apparently there had been a minor fender bender and the police were directing traffic around the area. Jim was impatient and drove right through the middle of it all!

Finally, it was a policeman's call to my daughter that put the spotlight on a looming challenge, taking the car keys away from Jim. Driving home from the museum one day, Jim drove into an area clearly marked, "no traffic allowed." A policeman witnessed the trespass and put on his lights coming right up behind Jim's car. Jim didn't stop. Siren came on. Jim didn't stop. Finally at the next intersection Jim stopped for a red light. The policeman got out of his vehicle, walked up to the driver's side and tapped on the window. He didn't give Jim a ticket, but somehow got our daughter's telephone number and called her. He told Karen that his own grandmother had begun having issues with driving before they took her car away and perhaps it was time for Jim to stop driving.

Almost everyone knows how hard it would be to give up driving—your independence is gone. You're stuck in the cul-de-sacs of suburbia. It was going to take an intervention to get Jim to accept the fact he could no longer drive. Friends, neighbors, and family all appealed to his good sense and that he didn't want to possibly hurt anyone. Finally he reluctantly agreed. We told him he could take taxis, that we would drive him wherever he wanted to go, that friends from the museum who lived in our area would pick him up on the day they gave tours (and they did), and that our grandson, David, would drive for him. But Jim never gave up asking if he couldn't take a driving class and then drive again…I think driving is in our DNA.

We did think it was alright for Jim to get his license renewed on his 80th birthday if for no other reason than to have an ID card. David took him to the DMV—usually a challenge for any driver. But as David told the story afterwards, the license was easily renewed even though it was obvious Jim needed help with every step of the process!

I would be remiss if I didn't mention two other human angels whom I know quite well: my grandson, David (DJ for David Jeffrey) and my friend, Toni. I mention them often in the emails. David watched his grandfather like a hawk and drove him wherever he wanted to go. He never complained about his grandpa's erratic behavior or requests, but gently guided him away from potential "pitfalls." In the same manner, Toni was a great friend to Jim, showing respect and caring no matter how difficult the circumstances.

I was a "bit" player in the unfolding human drama of this disease. Yes, the stress and continuing loss were mine, but so many wonderful people helped Jim and me, I can't imagine having done it alone. I give thanks for all the human angels, known and unknown.

Neighbors

… "And who is my neighbor?"

Luke 10:29

We live on a cul-de-sac with wonderful neighbors and writing this story wouldn't be complete without mentioning some of our traditions. For years we've always had a picnic on Memorial Day (to reconnect after winter hibernation); a picnic on the 4th of July, and one on Labor Day. We bring a dish to share and our own food to grill and meet in front of our house. Jim would put the grill out on the front yard and we always had more than enough food. Certain neighbors are known for their homemade salsa, some for their elaborate and delicious desserts, or home brewed beer. Not just neighbors came, but friends of neighbors or extended families of neighbors—a pleasant way to spend the day for those not traveling.

For years we've also attended each other's celebrations of life: weddings, confirmations, first communion, Eagle Scout award, special birthdays, and we've also mourned one another's losses, young and old.

And, if we really get snowed in in the winter, we've been known to make that an occasion too. I mention all this as our neighbors became part of our "informal" support. Jim could still participate in the social events. We were not isolated. Especially in the winter of 2010 when I wrote these emails:

12-21-09

Hi all; This has been quite a weekend weather wise, and I'm wondering how many other east coasters have been snowed in? It snowed all day Saturday and even though shoveling was completed on Saturday morning, it was to no avail—-another foot fell. Churches were all canceled which was just as well as no one was leaving our street. Last night our neighbor, Tom, who is an ordained Anglican priest, said he would be holding a service of Mass this morning and wouldn't you know it, everyone on the street came. Lara called me at 8:30 and asked what supplies I had as she decided to make Chili for everyone for after the service, so I found lots of goodies including a big box of Bagel Bites, a large can of tomato pieces, beans, and she was in business. Others contributed beer and wine. The service was so nice and the kids read scripture and Tom had a nice homily and communion was served—-not with the neighbor's wine—that was for later. Another person brought his guitar and carols were sung. After all that, everyone went outside and shoveled so that all the driveways were clear if not the street. Well, I haven't shopped or baked, but Jim commented on how nice the morning was and so we'll count the day as positive which it certainly was…

2-10-10

Hi all; It is snowing again but a caravan went to the store this morning and brought the food in on sleds… we have so much food in the house we could survive the rest of winter. The plow-bob-cat came this afternoon and all neighbors stood out in the driveways and clapped their hands and Johnny gave the driver a bottle of wine and I gave him a plate of fresh baked brownies…all this because when the caravan left for groceries, they saw this guy doing another street and promised him a plate of cookies if he did our street. We have never had our street so well plowed.

2-16-10

I forgot to mention that our cul-de-sac hauled a neighbor's wood burning pit out into the middle of the street on Thursday evening and we had a wonderful fire and roasted marshmallows which are wonderful with hot buttered rum. We also had graham crackers and chocolate bars. Did you know that 55 grams of chocolate consumed each week will help reduce the possibility of stroke? We are good for a week at least. Jim and I made it to church on Sunday.

Travel

Travel with a person who has Alzheimer's is not advised, but we did decide to attend the Antarctic Explorer's reunion in Madison, Wisconsin, in the summer of 2009. We flew to Milwaukee and my daughter, Patty, and granddaughter, Holly, met us there where we rented a car and drove to Madison. As we were walking into the hotel where the reunion was taking place, Jim asked me, "What are we doing here?" but the smiles and greetings of his former colleagues seemed to spark some remembrance and our visit there was special. I would not have made that trip, however, without Patty and Holly's support.

That fall though, we decided to attend the Navy/Air Force football game in Annapolis. Friends and family were there, too, and we've gone to these games for years and stayed with friends who live there. This time was different. Jim became very agitated and among other things, started walking up the street to "go home." He created quite a scene and before all was said and done our plans to drive up through New York to catch the colors of the fall leaves with my sister and brother-in-law had changed. Jim and I rode back home with other family members. A disappointment? Yes, but a lesson about traveling with Jim which we didn't attempt again. The noise, activity and crowds created an environment that was just too confusing for him.

We still went to church. Most Sundays though, he didn't sing the hymns anymore. I missed that as he had such a good voice (and had sung in the choir for years). Except one Sunday I heard him join in on a familiar hymn. Amazing what a gift to me a moment like that was.

PART II

Adult Day Care (The Rec Center)
May 2009 to June 2010

But his world, the things he loved to do,

were closing down…

Catherine Bergstrom

Finally Jim asked me to write a letter of resignation to the museum. His fellow docents and staff members had a farewell party for him and honored his work in putting together "a world class small library" as one commented. But his world, the things he loved to do were closing down. He didn't read or watch TV and wasn't capable of using his computer anymore. He could no longer even do the small chores around the house. He would sweep the driveway and front walk, and the neighbors made a special effort to visit with him when they saw him outside. Occasionally he and David would run errands or Jim and I would go grocery shopping or for doctor's appointments.

Then a tennis friend told me about Braddock Glen, an adult day care center run by Fairfax County, where her mother was a participant. I made an appointment to meet with Georgia, the administrator at Braddock Glen, and I liked what I saw. The building was spacious and comfortable. There was a sun room and, from there, entry to an enclosed garden. The lunch program, a hot lunch, was appreciated by all—staff and participants, and there were numerous activities all day. So, spring of 2009, I decided to have Jim attend at least two or three days a week. It was a great choice and we both grew to care for the excellent staff there.

The participants themselves were fun and seemed content. I have a picture of Jim in a Santa Claus suit handing out small gifts at the Christmas party, and he very much enjoyed all the various musical groups that came frequently—some high school groups included. There was always a puzzle being put together and usually a familiar favorite movie was shown later in the afternoon.

What really made Braddock Glen special was the quality of the staff—each one of them. They interacted with the participants in such an easy, pleasant way and enjoyed them as friends. Dignity for the person was maintained. It was not a "sad" place. I was entering a world I didn't know about and had not expected...the positive changes that were taking place for the care and support of those with dementia...and their families.

Though Jim only attended the day care center three days a week, those three days gave me a break. But Jim never adjusted completely to day care. He always felt he needed to "go to work." It was a particularly confusing time for him.

11-9-09

Yesterday we went to a concert—mostly country music—on free tickets from the rec center. Karen and David went with us and we were glad we didn't have to pay for the tickets as Jim only lasted half way—though he enjoyed it he said. Since the concert was at George Mason University, it was only 15 minutes from our house. Friday was not so good as Jim absolutely refused to stay at the rec center—everyone there tried to change his mind, but I finally took him home as he was taking so much time from the staff and he was adamant. I wish there were things he could do to keep occupied, but there is not.

11-10-09

Hi all; Today was perfect weather-wise, and I did get a few more bags of leaves ready for pick up. But it doesn't look like I've touched anything. And the leaves are still falling and will be for some time unless we get lots of rain and wind with the next storm. Jim went to the rec center without incident today—in fact he made the comment he had acted like a horses… It would be nice if he could go for a long walks, but his gait isn't too good, and the main reason he goes to the center is to stay active, involved, talking, and listening. They have music, play word games, watch films and have modified active games. People are there for various reasons—stroke, etc.—and they all become a rather close group. I notice everyone greets Jim and he responds.

11-11-09

Yes, we—staff and I—are surprised that Jim remembers his acting out in frustration. I think it is his soul that struggles to be free and speak. For me it is the hardest aspect of this disease to watch.

11-12-09

Hi all; It rained all day, but thankfully no wind—yet. I fear for the trees that might come down along with the leaves…and you should see the leaves: the street, yard, and walks are all a sea of yellow. Jim heard the weather report and wondered if he'd get left at the rec center—we wouldn't be able to come get him. I assured him that there is no river or stream between here and there. David and Jim went to Home Depot and the dry cleaners this morning while I ran other errands…they came back satisfied that they had accomplished all items on my list.

12-2-09

Hi all; Sorry for the lapse, but Jim has been having issues since Sunday evening and I think I've washed everything twice including bathroom floors, but that was not the worst of it—he was having so much pain that came in spasms. So doctor visit today, x-ray taken, and as David said, "The problem can be solved." You know the routine—everything our moms told us: drink lots of water, eat fruits and veggies, exercise, and some pills. Karen and David have been constant helpers and I am thankful. This afternoon after all had settled down somewhat, Daisy and I went out to do leaf raking…it was a sunny pleasant day, and I needed my 15 minutes of Vitamin D. I had missed my noon Bible study, and Jim missed two days at the rec center so tomorrow we look for a normal day.

12-4-09

Jim had the rec people call me to come get him early—I do not like the way he is walking or staggering is a better word. I hope he is better tomorrow after a night's sleep. It's impossible to get him to tell us what is wrong—he just does not respond in an intelligible way. He did eat a good dinner tonight. The weather

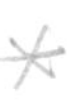

this weekend could get interesting as another coastal low is approaching, and the "S" word is being thrown around.

12-14-09

There was an open house party at the rec center last Friday and Jim had a great time as there was music and dancing and he is a good dancer. When I got there to pick him up he wondered who I was and where I was taking him. It's kind of been that sort of weekend. But he does keep asking when Patty is coming.

12-24-09

Hi all; Time to take a break from wrapping and the 5 million other things I think I should be doing—but I'm not. It is amazing to me how Jim is completely disinterested in anything having to do with Christmas—doesn't notice cards—we've received a jillion—presents—decorations, but he seems to enjoy the tree and lights…so strange. They did have a music presentation today at the center, and family kids came with the performers. He did enjoy that and the staff commented again today about his great Santa Claus act yesterday. I do miss him though.

12-28-09

Hi all; It is amazing how much energy, time, thought, preparation goes into Christmas and then how quickly the day is gone. I suggested that next year we go to some remote, warm place where our big decision is where to go to have dinner—no presents…we all have enough anyway. Jim and I did enjoy the evening service on the 24th and the music was wonderful.

1-12-10

Today Jim had his first of four treatments to coat his teeth to prevent decay…same treatment he had before…we go there at 8:30 and then to the rec center afterwards. He rebels about going to the center and  *the fact he never gets to do what he wants. He asked me tonight what I was going to do with the house so I said, "What do you suggest?" and he had a whole list of things he thinks I should do around here. He has great difficulty expressing those things, but I understood most of it. I reminded him of the things that got done this year—new roof, new lights in kitchen, replaced water pipe, new carpeting in his computer room, but of course there is so much more to do. It was good to have him talking in a somewhat rational way, and his frustration must be great. But his ability to do the smallest things is greatly diminished: fastening the seat belt in the car is becoming harder; finding his way to the bedroom requires assistance each day; he wants to help set the table, but can't get the right plates and utensils even when I tell him; he cannot tell night or morning. I don't tell these things to belittle him; it is just that he has been "robbed" of so much. However, he looks good and is quite sociable, and that goes a long way as people respond to him in a very nice way. I can only hope for as much.*

1-20-10

Hi all; No nap today so guess I'd better get my two cents in before I fall asleep—it being late afternoon. I went to the bookstore today to get a copy of The 36 Hour Day, *a book for caregivers, that was first published in the '80's and is in its 4th edition…I just heard about it from one of the nurses whose dad has Alzheimer's. Jim and I had gone to the commissary in the morning and enjoyed our shopping as few people were there…once I lost Jim but knew where to look…he was bagging up chocolate covered peanuts—his favorite. He didn't forget them or where they were in the store!*

2-1-10

David was over today and stayed with Jim this evening…who by the way is becoming more and more determined that he isn't going to the rec center any more…he said tonight that it is a free country! This from the same person who this morning said he was scared and didn't know where he was…I guess the good news is that he has no idea how much he has lost…conversely the bad news is also that he has no idea how much he's lost. It is very difficult to have a rational conversation with him.

2-2-10

I accomplished several mundane projects today—that is after I finally got Jim off—He refused to go so I just let him sit at the table looking at the paper and then I asked him an hour later if he was ready and he agreed. It makes me wonder if I'm doing the right thing by him. My alternative is to have someone come in here a few hours a day, but unless it were a former naval aviator, golfer, coherent type with a driver's license, I don't think it would work. Suggestions anyone? I feel as though I'm losing authority…I was throwing the ball for Daisy a few times this morning and finally said, "Last throw—we're going in" so she got the ball and sat down in the middle of the street—refusing to budge until I said, "Okay, one more time."

2-3-10

Hi all; Flash! It is snowing. Now you in Colorado probably wonder what's the big deal, but I want to say that it is a big deal here where the snow removal happens when the sun comes out and takes the snow away…could be days. Also, Jim absolutely refused to go to the rec center today. He was like a little kid—NO. It reminded me of the story his mom used to tell about Jim when he was a toddler. He would cry until he couldn't get his breath—scaring everyone in the process. One day he held his breath so long he passed out and Hildur—his mom—ran with him in her arms to the hospital a few blocks away. The doctor told her the next time it happened, splash a little cold water on his face. Problem solved…no more tantrums. So David came to my rescue as I had noon study today and it was a wrap up of the last four weeks and I also picked up my friend. Jim could have gone along, but he never wants to. An amazing thing happened…Jim asked David to help him order flowers for me, and so they did and afterwards Jim shook David's hand. As David said, "Grandpa was so pleased to accomplish something." 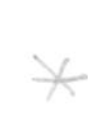

2-23-10

Hi all; News flash...the kitchen floor got washed today. Now to all hard charging types out there, this may seem very mundane, even pathetic, but truth be told it would be if it happened frequently, regularly, if there hadn't been the snow storms of the century with dog, guests, friends tramping through, all house-bound and satisfying their boredom by cooking and eating and we all know where that happens. Well that was two weeks ago, and still the unwashed remained unwashed...till today. Oh the beauty of it. Sorry. I just had to tell. Also took Jim for a pacemaker check today and that went well...working 90% of the time. Yes, it can take 100%...I asked. It has an energizer bunny.

3-9-10

Hi all; Lovely day today—sun shining—no wind—the ground is getting drier so we can start cleaning up all the branches and debris. Jim had an 8:30 appointment and that went well. Came home to walk the dog and play ball with her and then off we went to Costco to see what goodies we could find. We found plenty: coffee, wine, cookies, pansies (yes, colorful pansies in a large pot), shrimp, Ghirardelli brownie mix, some meat and to save ourselves, oranges and blueberries. Jim then wanted a hotdog and soda…why not.

3-19-10

Jim had had another "incident" which takes a while to resolve/clean and I'm wondering if he had a stomach virus which Toni now has? But he doesn't seem able to tell us anything about how he feels. He is "seeing" things like rain and wires and it is impossible to tell where that is coming from or what it means. They called from the rec center and asked Jim to come tomorrow—not his usual day anymore—as they are having dancing and they all know how he loves to dance. But first a lady from the continuing care center is coming to do an assessment. I've told her that Jim isn't ready to be there, but she feels it is better to have a plan rather than wait for a real crisis. He is starting to use profanity to express himself which is not like him, but I'd probably use profanity regularly, too, if I couldn't make myself understood.

3-22-10

I worked in the yard yesterday cleaning out flower beds etc. and was surprised to see how much is popping out…so soon after banks of snow had covered the ground. The lady from the care center came on Friday, and I did make a deposit for a reservation for Jim to go there, but am in much anguish about the idea…wondering why we just can't muddle through the way we're doing…would he be better off in that structured environment with activities just for folks with Alzheimer's? I just can't grasp the idea of it all. Toni and I are always surprised at what Jim remembers: last night we sat down for a very light meal and just began eating…Jim just sat there and looked at us and we asked what was wrong…He said, "Don't we say something before we eat?" So we do, and we said Grace and Jim ate.

4-30-10

I think I substituted a busy Thursday for the Tuesday's or at least today as Jim had his appointment at 8:45 and then I took him to the rec center…The appointment at the doctor's office this morning made me wonder what I'm failing to see. The doctor suggested assisted living for Jim as he said pretty soon his care will be overwhelming. His brain has taken leave of his bladder and notifying his stomach that he has had enough to eat. The thought of moving him is very difficult for me—as long as he is here things seem somewhat normal—there is also a sense of failure at not being able or willing to take care of him. He still gets up early for his breakfast—enjoys the dog—and church. Well there is a seminar on the 12th about when to move a person into assisted living—I've been invited to attend so I will. Both Patty and Karen are very supportive which helps a lot. Today at the doctor's a man came over to Jim and greeted him—this fellow is a docent and was on the library committee... but Jim didn't recognize him...or remember the committee. Well what did I read recently? Everyone has a photographic memory, but some of us run out of film.

5-7-10

Hi all; Jim refused to go to the rec center today as he had things he needed to do! A fellow from our church, retired Air Force and a docent at the Steven F. Udvar-Hazy Center, came to visit Jim today and they had a good visit—at least I think so as I worked on a project while he was here. It amazes me how this Alzheimer's affects a person…sometimes the simplest thing like getting under the shower head while showering is beyond him. I noticed the water was running quite a while and went to check…he was very upset as he couldn't get the soap off his face—so I turned the shower head on him and then turned him to face it…He was totally lost. I wouldn't have believed it if I hadn't witnessed it…One minute he is helpless and the next he's thinking he'll go traveling.

5-10-10

Jim was home today and mostly read mail. The other day I had the table set for breakfast and cereal and fruit out and then I left for a moment and when I came back down Jim had taken a dog bone from the bag on the counter and broke it up into his cereal bowl and poured milk on it and was happily eating. Oh my gosh! Lesson learned about leaving things on the counter.

5-28-10

Yesterday Jim and I had a very nice trip with a friend to the Steven F. Udvar-Hazy Center at the invitation of Mary, who was there to meet us at the door. The guards all smiled and came out to say hello and shake Jim's hand...he saw a few friends and we reviewed some of the aircraft and then had lunch where Jim ate a very large McDonald's hamburger—all of it. We also saw the very nice plaque in the library that was dedicated when he "retired." But Jim was very tired and confused last night.

By the end of a few months attending Braddock Glen, Jim balked frequently about going in, and when I came to get him in the afternoon, he was usually sitting away from the others, obviously not watching the movie or participating in games and activities. Alzheimer's was relentlessly isolating him, and now another symptom showed up...he became incontinent, bladder at first and then bowel also. Braddock Glen wasn't staffed for the kind of individualized care he was going to need. It was disappointing for me as it had been a good year with amazing support, not the least of which was the Alzheimer's support group monthly meetings I attended there.

Support Groups

You do not have to sit outside in the dark.
If, however, you want to look at the stars,
you will find that darkness is required.
The stars neither require it nor demand it.

Annie Dillard

For some reason being part of any support group had never appealed to me, but a friend encouraged me to attend an Alzheimer's Support Group. She said there were several in the area, meeting at different times and to visit various ones until I felt comfortable.

Braddock Glen had such a support group which met once a month and Georgia, the administrator there, facilitated the group. She even prepared a dinner for all of us each month and sitters were provided for the "participants" so the caregivers could attend. We met at 5:30, ate the delightful dinner, and then the meeting lasted one hour. Georgia is a thoughtful leader, very knowledgeable and experienced and she mostly let everyone talk and answered questions when asked. So everyone shared; stories brought laughter and tears; there were lessons learned: "home" is a place known only to the Alzheimer's patient (and is usually some place other than where they live); trying to teach a person with Alzheimer's how to do something is not possible (they don't remember the lesson!); understanding that respite time is essential for the caregiver—and encouraging one another to take that time away.

Honesty at the support group was the order of the day. One caregiver shared that when she learned her husband had Alzheimer's (eleven years ago) she thought "Oh, no, is he going to die?" Now her question was, "When is he going to die?" We all understood her question. It wasn't that she didn't love him, it was just unbearable to watch her husband of 54 years not be able to speak or walk or understand. He had once been a respected department head at a major university.

The caregiver's frustration was a topic at times as the comments and requests of an Alzheimer's patient seem so unreasonable. They could eat dinner and ten minutes later ask what was being served for dinner. We learned that the brain function that tells when the stomach is full no longer worked.

We learned that Alzheimer's—while a disease—has become a generic word for dementias with various causes. As brain research increases, doctors will be able to sort out the various causes and be more precise in their diagnosis. The bottom line for caregivers is that our loved one's "brain" no longer works.

Some of us have lost our spouses, but we still attend the support group as we listen and share our insights into the final weeks and months of care. Maybe most importantly, we survived and we still care and understand and want to be part of what is a positive light...that hour of genuine understanding;

of suggestions for whatever help anyone needed; of absolute non-judgemental listening; of knowing how lonesome one feels when conversation and sharing with someone we love just ceases—though that someone we love can be sitting across the table or the room—because talking or even remembering who we are is gone. It is hard to accept that. They don't look too different and sometimes they even have "good times" like rational thinking or speaking. I found those "good times" gave me hope, but with Alzheimer's it is a false hope.

Our support group has grown very close and Georgia wondered, and I agree, that our closeness and love and concern for one another developed from that shared meal sitting at a table and eating and visiting.

Some of us also meet for lunch regularly, our friendship is a positive, a blessing that comes from shared loss—a loss felt long before our loved one dies. We may come to our lunches bonded by the tribulations of life, but the banter, laughter, and chemistry of friends bring another bond: the joy and triumph of life. We call ourselves the "Deli Girls" as we always meet at the same deli, and one of our Deli Girls reckons our lunch is the equivalent of a $500 therapy session.

5-19-09

I went to a support meeting last Thursday evening and whatever set it off I don't really know, but the stories became hysterically funny and one just fed off the other until my stomach ached from laughter and my face hurt, too. The hilarity is of course the flip side of the great sadness/loss/turmoil we are all in. The masks came off for that brief hour as the stories of care giving that never were imaginable to us years ago were tossed out for all to share…and we all have shared in them. It is surprising that there are so many men who are "clients" at the rec center.

6-4-10

Tonight was a meeting of another type—the Alzheimer's support group and a good discussion by all. I'm coming to realize that maybe the move into assisted living isn't about whether I can take care of Jim, but how the family is scared that in the process of losing their dad they think they might lose me, too. Now I'm not sure that is something to be scared about, but I do remember our concern for our parents—it is a natural thing to do.

Time

The 36 Hour Day

Nancy Mace and Peter Robins

11-6-09

Hi all; I am happy to report that my new alarm system works—at least at 1:09 AM it went off and roused me from a sound sleep, and I had forgotten to just leave the "chimes" on and so the real alarm went off. When I finally came to and realized what was happening, I went downstairs and there was Jim, dressed, in the kitchen, and I sternly ordered him back to bed…. where he went as I think the alarm had scared him. So this is progress?

Caring for a person who has Alzheimer's becomes a full time 24/7 commitment. Their sleep rhythms are disturbed so that even night time may not provide normal rest. Then too, the caregiver has to make up for all the "errands" that two of you used to do. Jim had always been so caring, capable and helpful. I felt the loss even more keenly.

The following emails give just a small hint at my struggle to "keep up."

11-17-09

Hi all; another lovely November day…I could take a winter like this. Jim's appointment this morning went well, but took two hours as we had lab tests to take so he was a little late for the rec center. I came home to do a little cleaning after a busy weekend, get correspondence out, wash clothes, run dog, etc. I find myself wondering how I ever used to do things like sew, take classes, volunteer, raise kids, cook, clean, and all the extra hobbies I had while now I seem barely able to keep up. Time gets away from me—it goes so fast—literally. Am I that much less efficient? Poorly organized? Slower? Fussier? All of the above? I am going to call a couple of landscapers and get plans for the yard which will require: a green-scape, one that tolerates a big dog and lots of shade, but requires minimum work…I have ruled out concrete. I suppose I could also stop watching football, but not right now as it is time for the Monday night game. Love you all…

12-11-09

I believe my motto should be one I read long ago—"The fun is not in having nothing to do. The fun is having lots to do and not doing it." Oh, I just remembered I don't have the trash out. Too late… I would have to turn off the alarm, unlock two doors, open the garage door…forget it. Fun Fun Fun.

12-15-09

Hi all; Today Karen and I took our family wreath to Arlington and then I planned to make another attempt at getting the car registered….had all the paper work plus Jim's signature and his ID card and a copy of the power of attorney henceforth called the p of a. Well I needed the original copy of the p of a. I asked to see the person in charge and the Provost Marshall came out. It was an iron clad rule that the original was needed, but he gave me a one year extension on a sticker. But I came home and wondered about the rigidity of this military bureaucracy…spend 30 years serving your country—fly in combat zones like Korea—risk life and limb flying off carriers and then spend the rest of your life trying to get your car registered which I am beginning to see might be more stressful than being shot at by the enemy. Well then Karen and I stopped at the service center where I left the car for a check-up and got a loaner car in exchange. Then home to open the mail including a letter from the long term insurance—from now on referenced as ltc...which stated that they had received the days for Jim's day care—17 days!!!—he has 78 days. So I called the 800 number and pressed two and waited seven minutes to talk with someone who told me they had only received October hours...to which I replied..."Where have my other 6 proof of payment copies gone?" well could I hold while she asked the benefits person. More waiting... I would have to send them in she said...to which I replied..."What address would you like me to use?" and I read the letter advising me where to send these proof of payments—from now in referenced as p of p. More waiting and then a major apology as all papers had been received and someone—and these are my words—either from incompetence or laziness or indifference—had just ignored them as the exact days Jim was at the center weren't listed, just the number of days and the cost. To which I asked why I hadn't been notified that that was required—more apology. So I left to go get Jim and when I arrived at the center they had just gotten off the phone as the insurance company had called!!! I got home and put a pizza in the oven—and hoped it didn't burn. But the sun was shining today and the service center called to say the car was in good condition—a few smaller items they would repair. All for now—the football game is on…sorry for all my ranting and raving but it helps to do that.

Daisy

No man can be condemned for owning a dog.
As long as he has a dog, he has a friend.

Will Rogers

You, the reader, may wonder how a story about a dog, and one in particular, fits into our story. I actually wondered that myself when my daughter and close friend decided we needed a "companion" dog, and in fact, brought home for us an eight month old yellow Labrador whose family could no longer keep her. Our friend helped train her and she is a lovely companion. Jim called her "Sunshine" and when he moved to assisted living in June 2010 taking Daisy along for visits was almost mandatory. A few of our family emails tell about those visits.

I must add a disclaimer here as not all dogs respond well to Alzheimer's patients or their environment. Frank Fuerst's book, mentioned earlier, tells about the negative effect his wife's disease and related change of habits had on their dog. A family friend took their dog.

12-17-09

Daisy has been getting her walks most of the time, but at least many play sessions with the tennis ball every day. You needn't worry about her! She sits right in front of you…eye ball to eye ball…nudges your arm… drops her chew bone in your lap…waits for you to even twitch, at which point she eagerly jumps up and gives you the questioning look—are we going now? It takes severe hard heartedness to ignore that for too long…by which time you're beginning to feel negligent. She also looks at the clock—then you—then the clock for her noon lunch bone and at four for her car ride to go pick up Jim. Toni found that very scary that she seemed to tell time. The neighbors are also trained now—when they drive up the street to look for Daisy as we play ball in the cul-de-sac, though if she sees a car coming, she immediately sits down and waits for the car to pass or park. So it is funny to watch as the driver waits for Daisy to run and she waits for them to park. Well, time to take Daisy for a walk!

7-9-10

Daisy visited with Jim and Karen and David and was surrounded by 10 people—David said—who wanted to pet her. She stayed during lunch and did her Hoover thing.

7-20-10

This morning Karen, Daisy and I went to visit Jim and he was better…we sat in on the morning exercises which are good and then visited before lunch. There is one resident there who walks around continually—tall –thin…never an expression on her face… never seems to notice anyone or acknowledge them anyway. Today we crossed paths with her and she stopped, smiled and spoke to the dog and petted her. For that brief few moments, the woman looked very pleasant and personable…then the mask came down and she walked on. Daisy gets lots of attention at Arden Courts (assisted living facility), and everyone wants to tell us about the pets they had. Too bad they don't have a resident dog there.

7-26-10

Toni came by just after I got home from church and we went to visit Jim…with Daisy who is a crowd pleaser. Toni also was amazed at the response of the expressionless lady to Daisy. What part of the brain is it that allows someone to appear perfectly "normal", speak kindly, smile and respond to doggie kisses and then walk off with a rigid bearing and no response

to anyone or anything else around her? What brings

her out of her social isolation? What part of the brain connects? And why?

12-16-11

This afternoon Daisy and I went to visit Jim who was very happy to see Daisy as was most everyone else. Daisy is very good on these visits—I don't have her on a leash—she seems to know who wants to see her and then she lays down in front of Jim and just stays there.

12-17-11

I did go to church and visited Jim who was sleeping and has a cold and a rash, and when Daisy and I visited him on Friday, the dog carried on "verbally" in a way I've not seen. Daisy likes to have people recognize and talk to her.

12-20-11

I must mention that when Patty was at Arden Court with Daisy, a lady came and asked if she could take Daisy to visit her brother's room, and then asked if we would mind stopping in from time to time when we are there with Daisy. Many residents react very positively to dogs and Daisy doesn't disappoint if someone seems friendly.

PART III

Assisted Living June 2010 to February 2011

If knowing answers to life's questions is absolutely necessary to you, then forget the journey. You will never make it, for this is a journey of unknowables—of unanswered questions, inigmas, incomprehensibles, and most of all things unfair.

Madame Jeanne Guyon

Earlier in the year, our daughter, Patty, who lives in Colorado, acquired a list of assisted living facilities here in Fairfax, Virginia, and I called a few to make appointments to visit them, and then she flew home to go with me.

The three facilities we visited were all quite new and I was surprised/amazed at what was now the "accepted design" for Alzheimer's assisted living. Studies had been done at John's Hopkins to determine what the optimal surroundings were to reduce agitation and a sense of confinement for the resident. The result was a large usually circular building at ground level with wide well lit carpeted halls, large windows and doors to the outside secured area with a pleasant atmosphere and individual rooms with a bathroom.

We "dubbed" one of the three assisted living facilities the "chandelier" as the furnishings were quite elegant. It was also more expensive and a 30-40 minute drive from my home. I chose the one (Arden Courts) only a 10 minute drive away and it too was very comfortable…if one needed the kind of care they provided, as an assisted living facility is not a nursing home. The resident must only need bathing and dressing assistance and of course activities, food and a 24 hour secure environment. The cost is about 3/5 that of a nursing home.

We put Jim's name on the waiting list at Arden Courts. Mabel, the administrator at Arden Courts, came to our home to visit Jim and myself, and do an assessment. She felt Jim would do well in assisted living and commented that making the move before one was forced to—an emergency—was recommended. I wasn't quite ready for this but knew it was eventually going to be necessary. I turned down one availability in April but the pressure was on from family and friends to take the next step.

I just couldn't imagine placing Jim in assisted living; taking him out of his home he had loved, away from familiar comforts. Some days Jim was better than others and a hope would arise in me that he was going to be okay. Or a question; was it really necessary to place him in a facility? Couldn't I manage?

But the most daunting issue before me was telling Jim he would no longer live at home. I agonized about this for days, this huge change looming over our life together. One evening I just folded my hands and prayed, "God I know Jim is in your hands. Help me tell him and get him to understand." I still remember the sense of relief I felt and the tenseness in my shoulders slipped away. The next morning Jim and I were sitting out on the porch and out of the blue he said, "I think I should live somewhere else." I didn't say anything for a few minutes and then told him we had been looking for a better place for him. He asked, "Is it a nursing home?" And I told him, "No, and you will have your own room and bathroom." He went upstairs and came down with a plastic bag with two shirts in it and said he'd also like to take our son's leather chair. It was such an incredible conversation—especially as he wasn't able to talk much anymore—and then to lift such a burden from me. God's grace!

So in June 2010, Jim moved to Arden Courts and we were quickly caught up in the pleasant rhythm and caring staff and appreciated that time. They had quarterly seasonal parties for families and residents. Marie, the nutritionist, prepared great food. There were fun activities. I remember one Hawaiian luau party; flowers had been donated and volunteers helped make leis for everyone.

6-14-10

I guess the most pressing thing in my mind is wondering if I'm taking the right steps in regard to Jim… it is such an awful decision to make.

6-16-10

But the big news is I have changed the move in date for Jim to assisted living until Monday. Lots of reasons. Some I probably don't even fully understand except this morning I thought I would come unglued with all the things I needed to do before tomorrow and then I thought about Father's Day, and Patty coming to visit and she wouldn't get to spend even a day with her dad as they don't advise visitors the first few days after a move-in and adjustment period, and then I thought about my niece and how much Jim always loved her visits, and I thought this is crazy—why are we doing this this week?...So I asked the rec center if he could be there on Thursday and Friday and they said yes, and I called the assisted living center (hereafter referred to as AC) and told them of my change of date (I didn't ask) and then I took Daisy for a walk and felt like a ton had been lifted from my shoulders. To be continued...

6-17-10

Kind of a jumbled up day—guess that is what happens when you change plans.

6-22-10

The move has been made—rather without incident or comment. His room looked good as the girls had hung favorite pictures and he had asked for David's leather chair so we took that over. Also put the wings of gold—on a blue background—rug on the floor. Jim had that rug made in Hong Kong and it is beautiful—5' by 3'. My hope and prayer is that he will be happy or at least content in his new "house." As for me—I can't tell how I feel—relieved, shocked, empty…The days and months leading up to this have been so angst ridden that I thought I might fall apart. But the only emotion I felt this morning was anger at the facility as I was charged for three extra days as we put a few pictures in the room (not hung up) last Friday. I asked why his name wasn't on the door or his outside picture wasn't up if the room was his…they still aren't up. Then I looked at the poor unsuspecting administrator and said, "Oh, I know. This is a business." So the guilt ridden tearful wife they expected turned out to be some angry woman!

6-24-10

Jim seems to be doing okay (in the phone calls we've received from the center), but we can't visit him for a few days—or at least shouldn't they say. Meanwhile I keep expecting to see him in his usual haunts around the house—it will take time to get used to his absence. After taking Patty to the airport I was taking a different route home as the main road was a parking lot…I passed familiar landmarks and thought about visits past and was generally feeling a little down. Suddenly a small car pulled right in front of me with license plates that said, "It's Life." It did jolt me out of my reflections and I had to smile.

6-28-10

There was a family reunion in Minnesota which I really don't see myself attending…I'm in the middle of a sea change in my life. Not a death…not a divorce… but a loss none-the-less. I haven't even seen Jim since he moved in to assisted living as they ask family not to visit for a while. I miss his presence in the house. I don't feel settled about this move. I feel so sorry to miss this reunion, but my heart isn't in it.

6-29-10

I did go see Jim yesterday and they said it was okay… when he saw me he put his head down and sobbed… But I just hugged him and we went for a walk and then sat and visited…but his conversation was not understandable…He greeted members of the staff as they walked by and seemed to like them. The noon meal was cooking—roast beef etc.—and smelled delicious and so I walked to the dining room with him and then left as the meal was served. Other than his initial reaction—which they say is not unusual—he seemed fine. I told him I'd bring Daisy and he smiled at that thought. So we enter another phase in our almost 50 years together…one we wouldn't have chosen, but one we knew could happen. I'm thankful for caring staff.

7-12-10

Yesterday the assisted living facility—Arden Courts—had a Luau for residents and all guests, so Holly, Karen, David, Toni and I went. It was very well done with activities, music, and dancing, and very good food. Jim seemed fine and Toni thought that Arden Courts was all she had hoped it would be. This was her first time there. While there, I spoke with a lady whose mother has been a resident for three years… and the family has been pleased with the care. That is always good to hear. As for me, I keep seeing all of Jim's things…golf equipment…papers…suits and my mind hovers between seemingly unrealistic hope (for a brief moment) and then the pang of dismay.

7-15-10

I visited Jim. It was interesting. Jim has a friend and they walk around together holding hands so when I came to visit various staff came up to me and asked if I wanted to visit with Jim without his friend…I said, No, it's okay. As I said, I want him to be content with his new home…It doesn't upset me that he has a friend…what upsets me is that he has Alzheimer's. He seems happy to see me and holds my hand, too. Karen and I had to smile…she prayed for God's grace for Jim in his new home…we didn't know His answer would be a woman named Grace! Many of these folks with Alzheimer's are like lost souls or little children, searching for where they belong. The past, the present and all in between are jumbled together…if they find comfort I think it is a blessing…He has been slip/

sliding away from his family for some years now…if it weren't so, he wouldn't be in assisted living.

8-11-10

It is also really sinking in that Jim isn't going to come back—of course I knew that all along, but it wasn't something I thought about for any length of time. Well all for now…will shop and visit Jim tomorrow and have dinner with neighbors in the evening.

8-13-10

A rather quiet day today—but David, Daisy and I went to visit Jim who was not very responsive to us or even the aide when she came to get him for lunch…I did notice that he ate when we finally got him to the table. I did start sorting out papers in Jim's office today and have to go through them all as he has put together some unusual groupings; for example he had old tax info from RI stapled with a Christmas letter from a friend—long deceased—with a current monthly newsletter from the county with pictures of his mom, etc. There is also much interesting information on various aircraft that he accumulated in his job as docent, including a letter from a Japanese fellow who was on one of his tours and sent additional info. So I will turn that all over to a friend at church who is also a docent. Then there is much info on the Antarctic including personal letters—some almost in book form—that may or may not be of value. The last few years he was not good about acting on various letters or requests. He absolutely refused to let anyone help him so it just became more and more chaotic.

8-16-10

Still working on sorting Jim's papers with a little break now and then for church, the boys coming over last night, visiting Jim and of course, walks and playing with Daisy. I'm gaining a perspective on Jim's work that I hadn't put into a pattern before, but I see he was always in the forefront of projects; like being in the advance party for the International Geographic Year in the Antarctic; getting the street lights installed in the community; starting the library at the "new" museum by carrying (car load by car load) the books from the old museum to the downtown museum to get them registered into their system and then picking them up and taking them to the new museum, ordering bookshelves and library equipment along the way;

Starting a corporation with two others so they could get a grant from the National Science Foundation for a book to be written about Deep Freeze 1, then hiring a writer and helping her make contact with all kinds of people who were involved. Etc., Etc. He was not a scientist, or a librarian, or a historian, but he would get the ball rolling and then people helped. I am enjoying in some way going through all these papers as it puts me in touch with him.

8-17-10

I ran errands today and then went to visit Jim...he was in the community room and was the only one there, but great music was playing so we danced. He has always been a good dancer and they even have a great picture of him dancing so asked if they could reprint it in the monthly newsletter. He asked if I was alone and if I had enough money. It is amazing that deep down he is still concerned about his family when he has trouble speaking, eating and knowing where he is.

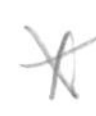

8-19-10

Also cleared out a couple of drawers which were a mess and I was looking for Jim's hearing aids which I haven't located yet. He doesn't wear them anymore as he was constantly taking them out and leaving them lying around and the staff at Braddock Glen finally put them in an envelope and gave them to me. That was obviously a few months ago…I took him for an audiologist appointment to see if they fit properly, etc, but he still wouldn't' leave them in…think I told you all that. But apparently the hearing aids only add to his confusion. So the search isn't critical.

8-20-10

Busy day today with a meeting about Alzheimer's—"looking in"—presented by one of the Alzheimer's Association staff. Karen went with me—it was at Arden Courts and Jim already had a visitor when we got there—a fellow from our church who is also a docent, and an Air Force fighter pilot. Guess I've mentioned him before.

8-24-10

I did get my hair cut this morning and then went to visit Jim. He seemed okay but was wandering around so we wandered together until I got him to go to the activity room and did the exercises with him. Then

I went into lunch with him and out of the blue he said, "I don't think I'm going to recover." It amazes me sometimes how much he seems to understand. I also had a few phone calls today and worked on the sorting out/throwing away process.

8-25-10

The Washington Post had an article today on finding a cause/cure/medication for Alzheimer's as the doctor says we will soon be overwhelmed with a tsunami of Alzheimer's cases at great cost to governments not to mention families. I leave you on that note.

8-31-10

I visited Jim yesterday and after a little visit, he said he had work to do and walked me to the exit! I guess that is better than having tears when I leave.

9-1-10

Daisy and I went to visit Jim and took some things over for him…he was sitting in the "living room" with several others from his "house" and all seemed very content. They really enjoy the dog.

One other aspect of Arden Courts that I appreciated were the speakers on Alzheimer's related topics, and one conference in particular called "The Yellow Brick Road of Alzheimer's" which was a talk giving details on the different stages of the disease. As the speaker very cleverly went through each stage, I thought, "Yes, Jim's been there. Yes, I saw that." Until she talked about the final stage and I realized that was where we were. Jim had begun falling for no apparent reason and had even fallen the week before. It was noted that these falls could result in a broken hip and then soon hospice was needed. Little did I know that Jim would fall two days later and break his hip. It was late September.

9-16-10

Then I was off to Arden Courts for a conference on Alzheimer's that was very well presented. If I were a nurse or someone needing to get accreditation, I would have received two hours for today. I decided that wasn't hard to take as we were also served lunch. So what did I learn? The ability to sign one's name is a big indicator of what stage a person is at. Also, I decided that one has to be like the new student in Psych 101…just because you have some of the traits of the subject in question doesn't mean you have the problem. I noticed a few people stopped drumming their fingers or swirling their pen when she mentioned fidgeting! Ha! Also I realized that Jim is in the end stages of this awful disease—that does not mean however that he is going to die soon as people can live years in this stage. I also learned that music is the last thing to go—it was probably the first we heard as infants...we lose abilities in the order we learned them. The other thing I learned is how extraordinary these caregivers are—these professionals...really dedicated. And last but not least—QTIP—which translates...quit thinking its personal. (That is their behavior toward you)

9-20-10

Latest from here is that Jim, who has Alzheimer's disease and a pacemaker, fell Saturday and broke his hip. He fell while he was walking in the outdoor area of his care facility.

While I can write about the hope I perceive with regard to recognition of Alzheimer's and day care and continuing care centers, one area that was very difficult to navigate was the hospital where Jim was taken when he fell and broke his hip. It may as well have been 30 years ago. This hospital staff (under staffed anyway) was not trained to care for Alzheimer's patients, and they would prefer the family caregiver provide a "sitter." Yet the hospital room—a double bed room—wasn't large enough for anything but the beds and bed side tables. One couldn't possibly put a chair in there. Also using restraints are not allowed. So the patient (Jim) who could not speak, did not understand he had a broken hip, and was in a confusing place, was given medication to keep him from being agitated. Trays of food were left at his bed though he couldn't feed himself or even swallow. They did move him into the hall near the main desk at night so they could keep an eye on him.

I remember standing in the hospital corridor and being told to make arrangements at a rehabilitation facility and do it quickly, and yet wondering at the same time if he could walk again, would he even know what the physical therapists were trying to do for him.

9-20-10

The break is in the bone below the ball of the hip, yesterday afternoon they did a 2 hour operation that uses 3 screws and a 3 inch incision to put him back together. As you might imagine this is debatable surgery on an 81 year old Alzheimer's patient who is unable to respond to commands. The other option was to continue sedating him (palliative care) but for how long? It was decided to patch him up and see where things go from there. I was relieved that they did the surgery.

9-21-10

Our—Karen and my—days are filled with visits with Jim. At night the staff puts him in the hall near their station so they can watch him as he has been so agitated. Today he was better but still wasn't stable—heart. Tonight, however, that was okay and he seemed aware of us and even ate. All kinds of people are coming to talk with us about physical therapy and best places to go for that kind of care.

9-23-10

We have decided to place Jim in a highly rated rehab center just for persons with dementia. It is 5 star rated and has a 6 month waiting list for senior living, but they called today and had a room available which they didn't yesterday. I don't hold out great hope that he is appropriate for rehab—he certainly isn't now as we can't even move him without great agitation on his part. Today was a zoo as everyone—hospice, care coordinators, nurses, were all meeting with us. Toni made dinner for Karen's family and me tonight and our neighbor went to visit Jim. Patty is flying in tomorrow having cancelled her long planned trip to MT with some of her friends. She feels it is more important to come visit. I did not ask her to do this, but know how she must feel. So tomorrow may be moving day for Jim—they transport him—if he remains stable. If he regains his ability to walk—with assistance—he can move back to Arden Courts, otherwise probably staying at his new place. I have a friend who is a social worker at this new facility and she knows what we are experiencing as her dad had Alzheimer's. Well that is the update from here.

9-24-10

Another day of much activity with our pastor, the cardiologist, the geriatric specialist, various nurses and Karen and then Jim was transported to the rehab facility at 7 this evening. He is having difficulty swallowing and is only fed pureed food and has to be aspirated from time to time. Patty arrived on time and

Toni picked her up. I guess I have to say that we were told that probably within a month pneumonia would overtake Jim. This is hard to write…but the decline is so rapid—the difficulty swallowing was starting to be noticeable yesterday at lunch—it is part of the disease. We were even questioning the rationale of trying rehab—just calling in hospice, but hospice is available where he is going and after 2 weeks if there isn't progress, that is what we will do. Meanwhile, visitors are welcome. So, we watch and wait and pray for peace for Jim.

Rehabilitation

Rehabilitation, learning to walk again, for someone who has broken a hip and had surgery, is standard and successful for those who are aware of their condition. Unfortunately, Alzheimer's patients are not aware—at least in later stages of the disease—nor can they be taught anything. They cannot remember from one physical therapy session to the next. However, a room at a highly rated rehab center opened up and we were "outta there" (the hospital) as the saying goes. On to the new facility though as I discovered as the days passed, the aides were not really trained or even seemed indifferent.

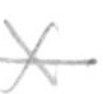

9-28-10

Patty and I visited with Jim several hours today and Patty went back this evening…she is not pleased with the care the aides give, and neither am I. But the professionals seem professional, and the grounds are lovely so we can go for walks. They have also solved the problem of his trying to get up and out of bed—they have a bed lowered to the floor and another mattress alongside so he won't fall. And though he can't make himself understood or understand or follow instructions or feed himself very well, he doesn't fail to say thank you when someone helps him.

10-4-10

Visited Jim. We struggle to get him to eat…it isn't clear to me why that is so, but it almost looks like he doesn't know how to eat or maybe he is too tired to eat. I will ask for some reasons tomorrow.

10-5-10

Sometimes one wonders…about what you may ask, and I can't answer. Harriet, Jim's sister who lived in California, died in her sleep last night. She wasn't ill other than the usual aches and pains of 84 years of age, and I know it was very hard for her to think of her kid brother struggling. They were very loyal to one another. So there is some schedule juggling going on, but this is a week of decisions for me to make for Jim. I talked with the social worker today and it appears they won't continue with aggressive physical therapy so a change is in order this Friday…we will have a conference about options then.

10-07-10

The biggest revelation we had today is the Jim is being given 3 different pain killers/sedatives and so we think we know why we cannot wake him up when he is sleeping which is often. I'm a little disturbed, but not surprised as response to our queries was slow... until today when questions were raised by an outsider.

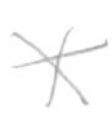

10-13-10

But the biggest news is that Jim had a very good day today—he gave me a big hug when I got there before lunch; he ate lunch by himself and didn't spill a thing and then when the physical therapist came into his room to do a few exercises—he was in bed at the time—she was going to show me how he sat up on the edge of the bed. She helped him put his legs over to the floor and then reached for the wheelchair to get him into it. But at that moment he said "no" and swung his legs back up on the bed by himself and lay down again. The physical therapist and I both spontaneously laughed and she commented that he could do what he wanted. It was wonderful to see him at least at the level he had been at Arden Courts—-though not walking. I know it doesn't sound like much, but days of seeing him so out of it was hard, and it was good to see his determination win out.

10-14-10

Over to visit Jim for dinner. He didn't eat too much and wasn't as alert as yesterday. I forgot to tell you that he got a haircut on Monday so I told him he was like Sampson—but different—he gathered strength from a haircut whereas Sampson...but he only weighs 10 pounds more than I do.

10-19-10

Meanwhile, Jim cannot speak except for a word or two, and he doesn't understand most of what we tell him and he is so thin, but now all the aides in the dining room are watching what he eats. He maintains his dignity in all this—hard as it may seem—doesn't complain by turning his nose at his pureed food, but managed to say—on a good day—cake and water. His liquids are thick so he won't drink too fast and pudding is not too satisfying as a dessert. I try to brush his teeth, but can't get him to open his mouth—he did "spit" today though and I practically cheered. So we're on a routine—up one day, down the next, and soon we will have to make a decision on placement... I'm not sure Arden Courts can care for him, but will let others tell us what they can and can't do.

10-20-10

When I visited with Jim today, the social worker—who is nice, but not too organized—said it appears Friday will be the last day for speech therapy so a change is in order; either as a regular resident where he is—not on Medicare—or move back to Arden Courts, which would be my preference. But it still isn't clear if Arden Courts can care for him though it has been under discussion for a week.

10-21-10

The plan for Jim is to move him back to Arden Courts on Friday along with a "sitter" and most likely hospice. The hope is that with more personal care, he could gain confidence to walk a little. While the care at the present 5 star rated place is adequate, it leaves much to be desired as there just isn't enough staff. David said that if they won't transport him, we will drive him as David said he could lift Grandpa into the car!

Return to Assisted Living And Hospice

And God who gives beginning gives the end...
A rest for our broken things too broke to mend.

John Masefield

Rehabilitation in the new facility was not successful. Jim couldn't learn and apply what he was taught to help him walk again. The speech therapy to help him swallow did seem to make a difference though. However, I had to make a decision: leave him at the new facility without Medicare (once physical therapy is no longer meeting certain goals, Medicare no longer pays) or move him back to Arden Courts where he would need a sitter. I decided to move him back as it was so much closer for me to visit frequently and the atmosphere seemed more pleasant. The sitter, who just happened to be available at Arden Courts, proved to be an exceptional young man, caring and patient. Jim introduced him once as his "assistant." Hospice now entered the picture as well, but in a limited role at first.

10-24-10

Hospice is setting up for Jim at Arden Courts by bringing in a special bed and wheelchair, as he meets the criteria they have for care, but he could rally as he looked very good today (some do rally)...the aide who will help Jim called today also and will meet us at Arden Courts. The floor manager at the rehabilitation center wanted me to consider leaving Jim as he has settled in very well and he is a nice patient to care for…she said they have a very good hospice there. Oh the pressure…and though I recognize that patients are in reality "inventory" for these care facilities, one hopes to make the best decision. As for caregivers giving out before their charges, it is easy to understand why: age is a factor as well as finances and the worry about that…statistics years ago said most people only have enough money to cover two - three months worth of care in a nursing home. Then there is the loss of the person and that loss goes on and on. I don't know if I will outlast Jim or not, but I have a few things mitigating for me…First, we bought long term care insurance long ago and that helps; Second, we had a living will in place and durable power of attorney so I wasn't second guessing what he would want or have to prove it; and, Third, and in my mind of greatest importance, is our faith and trust which calms the spirit.

10-25-10

David and I picked Jim up on Friday at noon and had no problem getting him in the car… he seemed to enjoy the ride, too. We got to Arden Courts and everyone greeted him and Grace cried. Maria, the nutritionist, fixed him lunch and brought a sandwich and chips for me and a soda for David as that was all he wanted. Oh, the speech therapist with whom I had an appointment on Friday before we left, never showed up—we were waiting and finally asked about our appointment. Finally someone came to tell us that therapy couldn't be given on the check-out day even though they knew we were leaving and in fact that was the reason the speech therapist wanted to see us so she could show me what to look for. Typical lack of communication in that place. Oh the hospice folks also showed up at Arden Courts.

It was good to have Jim back at Arden Courts, in his familiar room, and now he had a "sitter," Kingsley, a young man so perceptive and caring that we considered him a blessing. It was obvious to us that Jim liked him, too. The benefit of having Jim at Arden Courts, just five - ten minutes from where I live, was obvious and we settled into a routine of daily visits. The following emails reflect those visits.

10-27-10

Karen visited her dad this morning and was so impressed with the care he is getting…she had to give credit to Kingsley. Jim also looked at a clock and gave the correct time—speaking out loud!

10-29-10

I went to visit Jim today and he had walked this morning and is eating almost regular food. Kingsley wants Jim to walk with the walker and is trying to keep him out of the wheelchair. It is interesting to watch as Jim doesn't want to use the walker and Kingsley is no pushover. So it is a battle of wills, but I think it is good as it gives purpose.

11-2-10

Also today when I visited Jim they told me they wanted to have someone sitting with him at night as he doesn't sleep. They will try other meds first—checking with medical to see what might work. I think the current meds are having an opposite effect on him than intended as he isn't even sleeping during the day.

11-4-10

Jim was awake again last night and of course the concern is his falling again as he doesn't know he can't walk. Anyway, the doctor was in today and put forth a new prescription but I may still need to have a sitter for a while until a solution is found.

11-5-10

Also did a little shopping and talked with the Arden Courts people and I hired a night sitter as the medicine given to Jim last night—twice—didn't phase him. It was a new prescription. Both the nurse and I agreed he is going to "crash" one of these days.

11-10-10

Toni and I met at Arden Courts at 5:00 to visit Jim who, by the way, is doing very well and walked with assistance and a walker today. He looks good, too, and knew Toni and Daisy also. Amazing.

11-11-10

Meanwhile, Jim is not sleeping and poor Amy, the night aide, is trying to figure out ways to keep him from falling—he gets pretty agitated.

11-25-10

I went to visit Jim after lunch and he was in very good condition—he seems better each day and the sleeping pill David recommended—a natural product—is apparently working.

11-26-10

The sleeping pill is melatonin and it is a natural substance which many seem to know about and take… available in GNC stores—where David bought it. Funny how the natural stuff is the last thing they'll try. It pleased David so much that something he suggested helps his grandpa. And all of us who were in on the trauma of the broken hip from the beginning think we are witnessing something slightly miraculous. 'Tis the season.

11-29-10

Jim continues to do well, but is getting impatient about getting to work! I have to say though that he can't walk even with a walker without a great deal of assistance. And now with a hernia causing some swelling, they don't want him on his feet.

11-30-10

I also ran a few errands today and stopped in to see Jim as they had ordered oxygen today as his breathing was shallow this morning. But he looks very good, and everyone assured me that he was fine—just want the oxygen there and most every resident there has oxygen in their rooms. It is not a medicine—hospice brought it—just for comfort. He seems so content and calls Kingsley his assistant.

12-9-10

Tonight Daisy must have known I was going to visit Jim as she sat by her car seat belt, looked at me then it—several times in case I missed the hint. I couldn't take her to visit as I was going to the church dinner afterward. Jim looked good even though he fell last night—was not hurt. There are four hours when I don't have a sitter and I talked with the Hospice nurse about that. I almost feel that he must hate constantly having someone watch him. Comments?

12-14-10

I visited Jim during lunch today and there was music being played—specifically "Ave Maria" and I heard a gorgeous voice coming from the next table—it was the lady who just walks—never changes expression unless she sees Daisy. They tell me that before her condition deteriorated you could hear her sing all the way out to the reception area. Wow! Then you look around and realize the careers that are represented by the residents…nurses, doctors, state department, teachers—such a loss to family and community.

12-17-10

Will also visit Jim…they called today and are taking him off some medicine as his blood pressure is low, and a change in doctors so the hospice doctor is now in charge.

12-22-10

Today, Patty made peanut butter balls in the morning and all went to visit Jim. He seemed so pleased and when our neighbors went to visit him this evening, he remembered that his family had been there earlier.

12-25-10

So we had two wheel chair guests—Patty's mother-in-law and Jim. David and Daniel picked Jim and an aide up. All seemed okay. It was all spur of the moment as he seemed so alert when Patty and Darren (a grandson) and Daisy went to visit him in the morning that we asked the nurse (about taking him out) and she said, "No problem." Camille was here also, so we had 14. They stayed until late afternoon, and I thought it was the best gift. Jim is on antibiotics for a urinary tract infection.

12-26-10

Patty visited Jim today who was walking (with a walker) all over the floor. Kingsley is a wonderful aide and Jim enjoys the challenge of walking.

1-4-11

Speaking of coming apart, a good friend of Jim's visited the other day, and tears came as he was leaving. This friend was visiting in the area. It is very hard for some people to visit Jim.

1-5-11

Daisy and I went to visit Jim (and other residents) this afternoon, and all seemed good.

1-7-11

Jim has been very agitated and it took three aides—including Kingsley—to work with him, so a new medicine will be tried. I feel awful as one aide was hurt a little, but the nurse told me this happens...part of the disease.

1-12-11

But I had places to go...first to visit Jim who was totally asleep...couldn't wake him up...no response. He had been that way yesterday, too, and the nurse was checking him out...doctor called as we all think he was reacting to too much medication given for the agitation. So that has been cut in half. It still brings tears to see him like he was today...the emotions go up and down.

1-13-11

As for us, progress was made here as we got the tree out and went to visit Jim who was awake!!!

1-25-11

Our church is also doing a clothing drive this week and I've got many things to donate as the girls and I agree we should give most of Jim's suits away. They don't do anyone any good just hanging in the closet. A hard decision in some ways, but reality rules. Anything he could possibly still wear, I keep...I did get a call from a gal whose husband was at Braddock Glen with Jim and she is thinking of placing her husband in respite care at Arden Courts so she can visit her son, daughter-in-law and new baby in California. I strongly encouraged her as she is as reluctant as I was to place him anywhere.

1-26-11

Jim fell again this morning, but seemed fine when I was there...the minute someone's back is turned, he tries to get up.

1-28-11

I, too, wish Jim would not try to get out of his bed or chair, but one thing one knows about Alzheimer's patients is that you can't teach them...lasts about ten seconds. 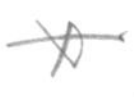

2-8-11

I spent most of the day at Arden Courts with Jim who is apparently slipping away...temperature, pain, no food or fluids and they called me this morning, but I was already on my way over. They are giving him morphine for pain...a suppository for temperature and various other things to keep him comfortable. I went over there tonight after dinner and he was sleeping and looked comfortable...and looked better than this morning so maybe he'll rally. Kingsley almost insisted I go home as he is stable for now. And there are stories of patients living three weeks without food or liquid as the pacemakers keep going! One of our pastor's came to visit and another one called this evening. The Hospice nurse was there quite a while and various staff checks on him from time to time. I guess it goes without saying that it is heartbreaking.

2-9-11

I had a dentist appointment today and then went to visit Jim. I wanted so badly to see him improved and was pleased that Kingsley had him sitting up in their living room. He even smiled at me, but still doesn't eat or drink. Kingsley gave him a sip of thickened liquid, but it just stayed in him mouth until it dribbled out. Maria, the nutritionist, asked me to stay for lunch which I did, but it was hollow as Jim just sat and didn't respond to food or his surroundings. Karen and boys came for dinner and they went over to visit Jim, but came away with tears in their eyes. Hospice was there today and another friend from church (Steven's Ministry). It seems as though everyone at Arden Courts is trying to help and mostly Kingsley who practically wills him to get better. No one can do any more. Patty may come on Thursday, but Mark is in California this week and next so she would only stay a few days.

2-11-11

Jim remains the same today and Patty is with him this evening though they also have a Hospice aide there. I have been looking at records for Jim's retirement/ discharge from the Navy and have copies though I'm not sure they are originals. I did come across some "official" pictures of Jim—starting in 1952 and then 1965 and 1968 which I think the girls will enjoy seeing. We have all been with him today at various times and friends stopped in to see him, too. We reminisced with some of the good stories of old that have been told many times, and we smiled and laughed at the memories, but Jim didn't seem to be with us.

The nutritionist sent Valentine cupcakes and bottled water for us. And so it goes...we can only wait, but he seems comfortable, and we are most certainly thankful for that.

All our family was with him Saturday night. Jeff brought his guitar, the Hospice aide was a gospel singer at her church and so we sang and probably kept everyone at Arden Courts awake except Jim. He died early Sunday morning on February 13, 2011. His face finally reflected such peacefulness; I could not wish him back. The girls and I sent out this last quixotic email to the family:

Captain's Log 2/13/11. Today I received a promotion which relieved me of command of Starfleet 8822 CHW to my able second in command and related crew. It has been a wonderful journey filled with memories that others couldn't imagine. I flew 41 combat missions in the far east; I've explored a vast continent inhabited only by penguins; I've commanded a squadron to train other Starfleet personnel; I've served in the command center where I observed firsthand the tragedy of Vietnam; I've worked for a car rental company where I had a great

ten years with some of the best sales people; and I've given tours for 19 years at the nation's premier air and space museum...But mostly I enjoyed a family that loved me and supported me...I will be in close contact, in my new position, with a crew member promoted 10 years ago...happy to see him again. I won't see the rest of you again for some time as my new post is in a different dimension, but as all aspire to get there, I'll be watching for you. Live long and prosper...

James H. Bergstrom, Captain, Starfleet

PART IV

The Challenge

Trust in the Lord with all your heart
And do not lean on your own understanding.

Proverbs 3:5

We caregivers often find ourselves second guessing the decisions we've made. Should we have placed our loved ones in day care, assisted living, or a nursing home? Couldn't we have cared for them at home? But there is no one right answer, everyone's circumstances are different, and the guilt we place on ourselves is an added unnecessary burden. We all do the best we can under stressful, extraordinary conditions.

As I mentioned at the beginning of our story, this isn't a "how to" book. I felt as though I "muddled through" a time of uncharted and unexpected behavior from Jim.

Yet I wasn't alone:

Our family offered absolutely solid support both for me and for Jim.

The Alzheimer's support group was a life line… invaluable in the information that was shared and the friendship given.

When push came to shove, as happened when Jim broke his hip and the question of the merit of surgery entered my mind, I called the Alzheimer's 24/7 Helpline—a resource staffed by knowledgeable professionals. The man I spoke with was knowledgeable and though he didn't tell me what to do, his information was correct (the surgery would be very hard for Jim). He didn't try to sugar coat the situation.

However, as I was muddling my way through and getting so much support, I realized the daunting challenge was for Jim. There were times of clarity for him and his strength of character and thoughtfulness (and even his sense of humor) were evident, even if for brief moments, to all of us who cared for him. His soul was intact while his brain and body betrayed him.

The doctors could not help him. Those who are and will be affected by Alzheimer's/ dementia need the support of medical research to find a cause and cure. That is about the only clear thing I really know about Alzheimer's; the challenge is before us, our society.

Epilogue

Now, with God's help, I shall become myself.

Soren Kierkegaard

Jim had requested, twelve years earlier, that he be buried with our son, David, at Arlington National Cemetery and so his request was honored though not until four months after he died. A burial with full military honors, which we wanted, waited its turn.

As for me, I was faced with seemingly endless paper work as dying doesn't go unnoticed by the government, or banks or anything that had Jim's name on it. It takes almost a year to settle it all, even with a will.

That first year, after Jim died, I attended a reunion of one of his Navy squadrons. Though I went with friends, I decided I wouldn't do that again as I felt Jim's absence even more keenly.

I have continued attending the Alzheimer's support group once a month—actually three of us who lost spouses to Alzheimer's continue to attend. We are able to be supportive, and what's more, we survived.

I was surprised at how quickly the difficult times of Jim's Alzheimer's became a distant memory and I could remember all the good years we enjoyed together. Someone once wrote that when remembering the loss of a loved one, there are two kinds of memory; the reason for the loss (illness, accident) and the memory before life went awry where eventually we become "keepers of the memory," those times that bring a smile of remembrance…if also the sharp twang of loss.

Now it is up to me and that takes adjusting, too. It is easy to wonder what my purpose can be. I'm not a wife/caregiver anymore, but I look around at all there is to do, and soon the issue becomes one of focus. I enjoy my Bible study group, church, the Deli Girls, Daisy and her walks, my house and yard, travel to visit friends and family, exercise classes, my grandchildren and their parents, Sudoku, the weather channel, daily family emails and friends.

Each morning I thank God for the day and for His Grace, which is sufficient for me. (2 Corinthians 12:9). I leave you, the reader, with one of my favorite verses:

> *Now to Him who is able to do far more abundantly beyond all that we ask or think, according to the power that works within us, to Him be the glory in the church and in Christ Jesus to all generations forever and ever. Amen.*
>
> Ephesians 3:20-21

Bibliography

Buechner, Frederich. *The Sacred Journey.* San Fransisco: Harper & Row, 1982. Print.

Dillard, Annie. *Teaching a Stone to Talk: Expeditions and Encounters.* New York: Haper & Row, 1982. Print.

Fuerst, Frank. *Alzheimer's Care with Dignity.* Warrenton, VA: F. Fuerst, 2007. Print.

Guyon, Madame Jeanne. *Spiritual Torrents.* Augusta, Maine: Christian Books, 1984. Print.

Kierkegaard, Søren, and Perry D. LeFevre. *The Prayers of Kierkegaard.* Chicago: University of Chicago, 1996. Print.

Mace, Nancy L., and Peter V. Rabins. *The 36-hour Day: A Family Guide to Caring for People with Alzheimer Disease, Other Dementias, and Memory Loss in Later Life.* Baltimore: Johns Hopkins UP, 2006. Print.

Masefield, John. *The Everlasting Mercy and the Widow in the Bye Street*. New York: Macmillan, 1916. Print.

Rogers, Will, and Joseph H. Carter. *Never Met a Man I Didn't Like: The Life and Writings of Will Rogers*. New York: Avon, 1991. Print.

CPSIA information can be obtained at www.ICGtesting.com
Printed in the USA
BVOW031916250413

319153BV00001B/85/P